I0114765

This journal was created by Millie Rose in hopes of sparking a little magic and joy into your everyday life. Through practicing positive affirmations, daily gratitude and a few little wellness rituals along the way, to have you loving yourself and kicking those life goals in no time.

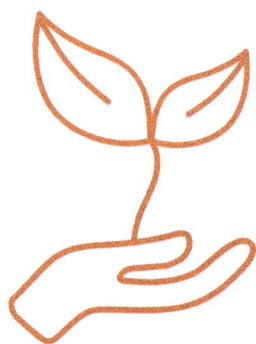

This journal

belongs to:

_____

What is Gratitude?

- Being aware of and thankful for the amazing things and/or people you already have in your life.
- By expressing thanks for all that you have; you shift your mindset from being hungry for change to feeling satisfied with what you already have. Once you believe you have enough you are open to receiving more and more and more.
- A positive emotion that gives you feelings of pure happiness and joy - that warm and fuzzy feeling.
- Filling you with love and appreciation.

Benefits of Gratitude:

- Helps you stay grounded.
- Improves mental health.
- Boosts the immune system.
- Better sleep.
- Reduces stress levels, increases happiness & positivity.
- Improves relationships.
- Can lead to self-improvement, supporting you to achieve your goals.
- Cultivating a sense of gratitude supports your overall health and well-being and can even lower blood pressure.

These are just a few examples of some of the amazing benefits of practicing gratitude regularly.

What are Positive Affirmations?

- Empowering words or phrases that we repeat to ourselves that state you already are or have what you desire. e.g. "I am open to learning and growth, and I WILL succeed", "I AM PHENOMENAL".
- The practice of positive thinking and kind self-talk which makes us feel good, reshaping the way we see ourselves in a much more positive light.

Benefits of Positive Affirmations:

- Reduces anxiety.
- Improves mood.
- Enhances self-esteem.
- The mind works through repetition, so by repeating positive affirmations, you are rewiring your brain, to form those new positive neural pathways and replace negative thought patterns with positive affirmations, to create a new positive belief.
- Even if this may feel uncomfortable to begin with, you may not believe what you are affirming, BUT the more you repeat these positive affirmations, your unconscious mind WILL program your brain to believe them.
- If you can program your brain to believe you can't do something, then you can reprogram your brain to believe you CAN!
- The power comes from within.
- Speak kindly to yourself and watch yourself grow.
    In case you didn't know...**YOU ARE AMAZING!!**

Self-Care Rituals

Self-care is an act to take care of your physical, emotional and mental wellbeing.

Now, what this looks like can differ from person to person. Below are just a few examples of some self-care rituals you can incorporate into your everyday life.

- Meditation- just a few minutes of meditation can calm you, relieve stress, boost your immune system and help to prevent and manage chronic disease.
- Tea-time- there are many different teas that can support your immune system, for example Peppermint tea can relieve tension headaches and migraines, and Camomile tea can reduce inflammation, anxiety and promote sleep.
- 10/10/10 ritual- everyday spend 10minutes in nature, 10minutes of movement and 10minutes of stillness/meditation.
- Morning cacao- try replacing your morning coffee with a warm glass of cacao- in a saucepan choose your desired milk with 1-2 tablespoon of cacao, a dash of maple syrup - rich in minerals and antioxidants. This will give you energy without the coffee crash you can experience.

Self-Care Rituals

- Have a lazy day - relax, watch a movie and don't feel guilty about it.
- Declutter your home or workspace - this can reduce stress, making you feel calmer and more in control.
- Commit to your skincare routine & wear your sunscreen - you'll thank me later.
- Stay connected with friends and loved ones.
- Go for a walk or surf, do yoga, paint, read a book, fuel your body with wholesome foods.
- Listen to your favorite song and dance like no one's watching.
- Relax in the bath with some essential oils.
- Get out & explore - do something that makes you feel ALIVE.
- Switch off your phone for an hour of the day.
- Have a laugh - laughter decreases stress hormones and increases endorphins.
- Slow down, listen to your body & stay hydrated!
- AND last but not least use your gratitude journal EVERYDAY!!!

Now have a think about what makes YOU feel good? What feeds your soul? What does self-care look like for you? Throughout the course of this journal, you will be prompted to include one self-care ritual each week.

My Gratitude Journal Intentions!

What would I like to achieve from practicing gratitude?

_____

_____

_____

What would this allow me?

_____

_____

_____

What are my goals and aspirations in life right now?

_____

_____

_____

What are 3 things I'm willing to do to bring me closer to my goals?

_____

_____

_____

My Values!

Below I would like you to write down your core values when it comes to family & friends, money & finance, health, work & career:

Family & Friends

_____

_____

_____

Money & Finance

_____

_____

_____

Health

_____

_____

_____

Work & Career

_____

_____

_____

<u>Week 1</u>

This week's self-care ritual:

_____
_____
_____
_____

This week I aspire to:

_____
_____
_____
_____

What inspires me to stay focused and motivated?

_____
_____
_____
_____

What do I LOVE most about myself this week?

Date: / /
3 Things I am Grateful for:

1-

_____
_____
_____
_____

2-

_____
_____
_____
_____

3-

_____
_____
_____
_____

Positive Affirmation of the Day:

_____

Thoughts/feelings to let go of:

_____
_____
_____

Date: /   /

3 Things I am Grateful for:

1-

_____
_____
_____
_____

2-

_____
_____
_____
_____

3-

_____
_____
_____
_____

Positive Affirmation of the Day:

_____

Thoughts/feelings to let go of:

_____
_____
_____

Date: / /

3 Things I am Grateful for:

1-

_____

_____

_____

_____

2-

_____

_____

_____

_____

3-

_____

_____

_____

_____

Positive Affirmation of the Day:

_____

Thoughts/feelings to let go of:

_____

_____

_____

3 Things I am Grateful for:

1-

_____
_____
_____
_____

2-

_____
_____
_____

3-

_____
_____
_____
_____

Positive Affirmation of the Day:

_____

Thoughts/feelings to let go of:

_____
_____
_____

Date: /   /

3 Things I am Grateful for:

1-

_____

_____

_____

_____

2-

_____

_____

_____

_____

3-

_____

_____

_____

_____

Positive Affirmation of the Day:

_____

Thoughts/feelings to let go of:

_____

_____

_____

Date: /   /

3 Things I am Grateful for:

1-

_____
_____
_____
_____

2-

_____
_____
_____
_____

3-

_____
_____
_____
_____

Positive Affirmation of the Day:

_____

Thoughts/feelings to let go of:

_____
_____
_____

Date: /   /

3 Things I am Grateful for:

1-

_____
_____
_____
_____

2-

_____
_____
_____
_____

3-

_____
_____
_____
_____

Positive Affirmation of the Day:

_____

Thoughts/feelings to let go of:

_____
_____
_____

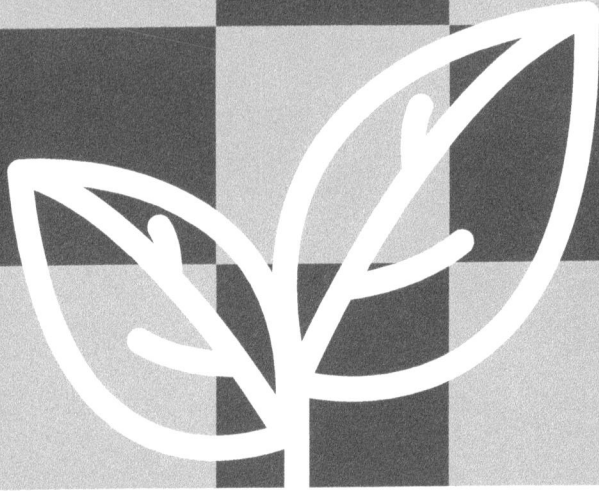

Youth
has
no
age

-Pablo Picasso

Week 2

This week's self-care ritual:

_____

_____

_____

_____

This week I aspire to:

_____

_____

_____

_____

What am I looking forward to most this week?

_____

_____

_____

_____

What do I LOVE most about myself this week?

Date: / /

3 Things I am Grateful for:

1-

_____

_____

_____

_____

2-

_____

_____

_____

_____

3-

_____

_____

_____

_____

Positive Affirmation of the Day:

_____

Thoughts/feelings to let go of:

_____

_____

_____

Date: /   /

3 Things I am Grateful for:

1-

_____

_____

_____

_____

2-

_____

_____

_____

_____

3-

_____

_____

_____

_____

Positive Affirmation of the Day:

_____

Thoughts/feelings to let go of:

_____

_____

_____

Date: /   /

3 Things I am Grateful for:

1-

_____

_____

_____

_____

2-

_____

_____

_____

_____

3-

_____

_____

_____

_____

Positive Affirmation of the Day:

_____

Thoughts/feelings to let go of:

_____

_____

Date: /   /

3 Things I am Grateful for:

1-

_____

_____

_____

_____

2-

_____

_____

_____

_____

3-

_____

_____

_____

_____

Positive Affirmation of the Day:

_____

Thoughts/feelings to let go of:

_____

_____

_____

Date: /   /
3 Things I am Grateful for:

1-

_____
_____
_____
_____

2-

_____
_____
_____
_____

3-

_____
_____
_____
_____

Positive Affirmation of the Day:

_____

Thoughts/feelings to let go of:

_____
_____
_____

3 Things I am Grateful for:

1-

_____
_____
_____
_____

2-

_____
_____
_____
_____

3-

_____
_____
_____
_____

Positive Affirmation of the Day:

_____

Thoughts/feelings to let go of:

_____
_____
_____

3 Things I am Grateful for:

1-

_____

2-

_____

3-

_____

Positive Affirmation of the Day:

_____

Thoughts/feelings to let go of:

_____

Fun Fact:
Cashews are known to be a natural source for boosting mood. Cashews contain mood-stabilizing vitamins: B6, magnesium, niacin, and tryptophan which converts to serotonin - the feel-good hormone.

Week 3

This week's self-care ritual:

_____
_____
_____
_____

This week I aspire to:

_____
_____
_____
_____

What are my favourite meals I enjoy eating and cooking?

_____
_____
_____
_____

What do I LOVE most about myself this week?

Date: /   /

3 Things I am Grateful for:

1-

_____
_____
_____
_____

2-

_____
_____
_____
_____

3-

_____
_____
_____
_____

Positive Affirmation of the Day:

_____

Thoughts/feelings to let go of:

_____
_____
_____

Date: / /
3 Things I am Grateful for:

1-
_____
_____
_____
_____

2-
_____
_____
_____
_____

3-
_____
_____
_____
_____

Positive Affirmation of the Day:
_____

Thoughts/feelings to let go of:
_____
_____
_____

Date: / /

3 Things I am Grateful for:

1-

_____

_____

_____

_____

2-

_____

_____

_____

_____

3-

_____

_____

_____

_____

Positive Affirmation of the Day:

_____

Thoughts/feelings to let go of:

_____

_____

_____

Date: / /

3 Things I am Grateful for:

1-

_____
_____
_____
_____

2-

_____
_____
_____
_____

3-

_____
_____
_____
_____

Positive Affirmation of the Day:

_____

Thoughts/feelings to let go of:

_____
_____
_____

Date: /   /

3 Things I am Grateful for:

1-

_____

_____

_____

_____

2-

_____

_____

_____

_____

3-

_____

_____

_____

_____

Positive Affirmation of the Day:

_____

Thoughts/feelings to let go of:

_____

_____

_____

Date: /   /

3 Things I am Grateful for:

1-

_____

_____

_____

_____

2-

_____

_____

_____

3-

_____

_____

_____

_____

Positive Affirmation of the Day:

_____

Thoughts/feelings to let go of:

_____

_____

_____

Date: / /
3 Things I am Grateful for:

1-

_____
_____
_____
_____

2-

_____
_____
_____
_____

3-

_____
_____
_____
_____

Positive Affirmation of the Day:

_____

Thoughts/feelings to let go of:

_____
_____
_____

ALLOW YOUR PASSION TO BECOME YOUR PURPOSE,
AND IT WILL ONE DAY, BECOME YOUR PROFESSION.

-UNKNOWN

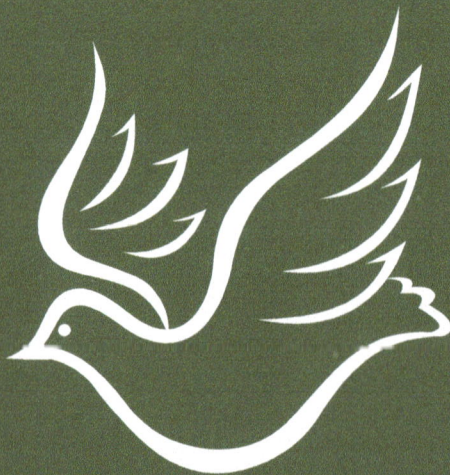

<u>Week 4</u>

This week's self-care ritual:

_____
_____
_____
_____

This week I aspire to:

_____
_____
_____
_____

What are my passions?

_____
_____
_____
_____

What do I LOVE most about myself this week?

3 Things I am Grateful for:

1-

_____
_____
_____
_____

2-

_____
_____
_____
_____

3-

_____
_____
_____
_____

Positive Affirmation of the Day:

_____

Thoughts/feelings to let go of:

_____
_____
_____

Date: / /
3 Things I am Grateful for:

1-

_____

_____

_____

_____

2-

_____

_____

_____

_____

3-

_____

_____

_____

_____

Positive Affirmation of the Day:

_____

Thoughts/feelings to let go of:

_____

_____

_____

Date: /   /

3 Things I am Grateful for:

1-

_____

_____

_____

_____

2-

_____

_____

_____

_____

3-

_____

_____

_____

_____

Positive Affirmation of the Day:

_____

Thoughts/feelings to let go of:

_____

_____

_____

Date: /   /

3 Things I am Grateful for:

1-

_____
_____
_____
_____

2-

_____
_____
_____
_____

3-

_____
_____
_____
_____

Positive Affirmation of the Day:

_____

Thoughts/feelings to let go of:

_____
_____
_____

Date: /   /
3 Things I am Grateful for:

1-

_____
_____
_____
_____

2-

_____
_____
_____
_____

3-

_____
_____
_____
_____

Positive Affirmation of the Day:

_____

Thoughts/feelings to let go of:

_____
_____
_____

Date: /   /

3 Things I am Grateful for:

1-

_____

_____

_____

_____

2-

_____

_____

_____

_____

3-

_____

_____

_____

_____

Positive Affirmation of the Day:

_____

Thoughts/feelings to let go of:

_____

_____

_____

3 Things I am Grateful for:

1-

_____

_____

_____

_____

2-

_____

_____

_____

_____

3-

_____

_____

_____

_____

Positive Affirmation of the Day:

_____

Thoughts/feelings to let go of:

_____

_____

_____

Chia Pudding Recipe-

Ingredients:
- 2 tablespoons of chia seeds
- 1/4 cup of unsalted cashew nuts
- blueberries
- banana
- cacao nibs
- cinnamon
- maple syrup

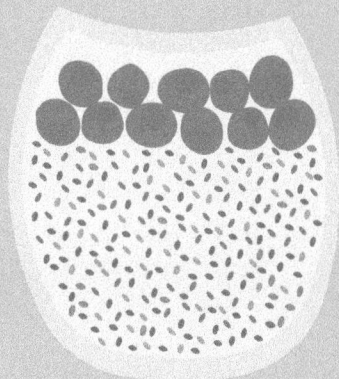

Method:
1- To make the cashew milk, use 1/4 cup of cashews to 2 cups of water, a dash of salt, blend and sieve to desired consistency.
2- Add chia seeds to 1 cup of cashew milk with a dash of maple syrup, refrigerate overnight.
3-Top chia pudding with blueberries, banana, cacao nibs, cinnamon and a dash of maple syrup to serve.

Benefits:
Anti-ageing, full of antioxidants, anti-inflammatory, fibre, omega-3, minerals, rich in protein and our favourite - this chia pudding is packed with mood boosting properties AND it's delicious.

Week 5

This week's self-care ritual:

_____

_____

_____

_____

This week I aspire to:

_____

_____

_____

_____

If I could have any job in the world what would it be?

_____

_____

_____

What do I LOVE most about myself this week?

Date: / /

3 Things I am Grateful for:

1-

_____
_____
_____
_____

2-

_____
_____
_____
_____

3-

_____
_____
_____
_____

Positive Affirmation of the Day:

_____

Thoughts/feelings to let go of:

_____
_____
_____

Date: / /
3 Things I am Grateful for:

1-

_____
_____
_____
_____

2-

_____
_____
_____
_____

3-

_____
_____
_____
_____

Positive Affirmation of the Day:

_____

Thoughts/feelings to let go of:

_____
_____
_____

Date: /   /

3 Things I am Grateful for:

1-

_____

_____

_____

_____

2-

_____

_____

_____

_____

3-

_____

_____

_____

_____

Positive Affirmation of the Day:

_____

Thoughts/feelings to let go of:

_____

_____

_____

Date: / /
3 Things I am Grateful for:

1-

_____

_____

_____

_____

2-

_____

_____

_____

3-

_____

_____

_____

_____

Positive Affirmation of the Day:

_____

Thoughts/feelings to let go of:

_____

_____

_____

Date: / /
3 Things I am Grateful for:

1-

_____
_____
_____
_____

2-

_____
_____
_____
_____

3-

_____
_____
_____
_____

Positive Affirmation of the Day:

_____

Thoughts/feelings to let go of:

_____
_____
_____

3 Things I am Grateful for:

1-

_____
_____
_____
_____

2-

_____
_____
_____
_____

3-

_____
_____
_____
_____

Positive Affirmation of the Day:

_____

Thoughts/feelings to let go of:

_____
_____
_____

Date: / /

3 Things I am Grateful for:

1-

_____

_____

_____

_____

2-

_____

_____

_____

_____

3-

_____

_____

_____

_____

Positive Affirmation of the Day:

_____

Thoughts/feelings to let go of:

_____

_____

_____

Mushrooms!

Mushrooms are packed with essential vitamins, minerals & antioxidants!

Rich in calcium, protein, iron, copper, and magnesium!

It's best to include a variety of different mushrooms within your diet to really gain the full health benefits.

- Source of Vitamin D - organic mushrooms will have a higher source of Vitamin D to supermarket mushrooms.
- Anti-aging - yes you heard right - Mushrooms contain antioxidants that neutralise the free radicals and can stop or delay damage to cells, reducing the aging process.
- Promote lower cholesterol.
- Lower blood pressure.
- Boost immune system - with anti-inflammatory properties.
- Good for gut health- source of prebiotic.
- Support brain health & memory.

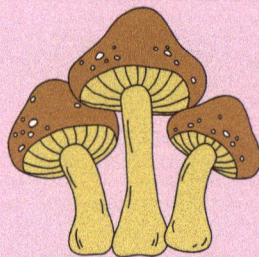

__Week 6__

This week's self-care ritual:

_____
_____
_____
_____

This week I aspire to:

_____
_____
_____
_____

Name one goal I want to achieve?

_____
_____
_____
_____

What do I LOVE most about myself this week?

Date: /   /

3 Things I am Grateful for:

1-

_____

_____

_____

_____

2-

_____

_____

_____

_____

3-

_____

_____

_____

_____

Positive Affirmation of the Day:

_____

Thoughts/feelings to let go of:

_____

_____

_____

Date: /   /

3 Things I am Grateful for:

1-

2-

3-

Positive Affirmation of the Day:

Thoughts/feelings to let go of:

Date: /   /

3 Things I am Grateful for:

1-

_____
_____
_____
_____

2-

_____
_____
_____
_____

3-

_____
_____
_____
_____

Positive Affirmation of the Day:

_____

Thoughts/feelings to let go of:

_____
_____
_____

Date: / /

3 Things I am Grateful for:

1-

_____

_____

_____

_____

2-

_____

_____

_____

_____

3-

_____

_____

_____

_____

Positive Affirmation of the Day:

_____

Thoughts/feelings to let go of:

_____

_____

_____

Date: / /
3 Things I am Grateful for:

1-

_____
_____
_____
_____

2-

_____
_____
_____
_____

3-

_____
_____
_____
_____

Positive Affirmation of the Day:

_____

Thoughts/feelings to let go of:

_____
_____
_____

Date: / /
3 Things I am Grateful for:

1-

_____

_____

_____

_____

2-

_____

_____

_____

_____

3-

_____

_____

_____

_____

Positive Affirmation of the Day:

_____

Thoughts/feelings to let go of:

_____

_____

_____

Date: /   /

3 Things I am Grateful for:

1-

_____

_____

_____

_____

2-

_____

_____

_____

_____

3-

_____

_____

_____

_____

Positive Affirmation of the Day:

_____

Thoughts/feelings to let go of:

_____

_____

_____

Fun Fact:
Taking in 5 deep abdominal breaths before eating, tricks the body into thinking it's not stressed, and kick starts metabolism, so your body doesn't produce cortisol.

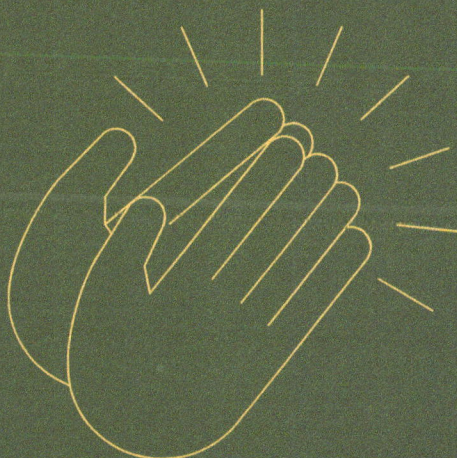

__Week 7__

This week's self-care ritual:

_____

_____

_____

_____

This week I aspire to:

_____

_____

_____

_____

What is one step I can take this week to move
closer to my goal?

_____

_____

_____

_____

What do I LOVE most about myself this week?

Date: /   /

3 Things I am Grateful for:

1-

_____
_____
_____
_____

2-

_____
_____
_____
_____

3-

_____
_____
_____
_____

Positive Affirmation of the Day:

_____

Thoughts/feelings to let go of:

_____
_____
_____

Date: /   /

3 Things I am Grateful for:

1-

_____

_____

_____

_____

2-

_____

_____

_____

_____

3-

_____

_____

_____

_____

Positive Affirmation of the Day:

_____

Thoughts/feelings to let go of:

_____

_____

_____

Date: /   /

3 Things I am Grateful for:

1-

2-

3-

Positive Affirmation of the Day:

Thoughts/feelings to let go of:

Date: / /
3 Things I am Grateful for:

1-

_____
_____
_____
_____

2-

_____
_____
_____
_____

3-

_____
_____
_____
_____

Positive Affirmation of the Day:

_____

Thoughts/feelings to let go of:

_____
_____
_____

Date: /   /

3 Things I am Grateful for:

1-

_____
_____
_____
_____

2-

_____
_____
_____
_____

3-

_____
_____
_____
_____

Positive Affirmation of the Day:

_____

Thoughts/feelings to let go of:

_____
_____
_____

Date: /   /

3 Things I am Grateful for:

1-

_____
_____
_____
_____

2-

_____
_____
_____
_____

3-

_____
_____
_____
_____

Positive Affirmation of the Day:

_____

Thoughts/feelings to let go of:

_____
_____
_____

Date: / /
3 Things I am Grateful for:

1-

_____
_____
_____

_____

2-

_____
_____
_____

_____

3-

_____
_____
_____

_____

Positive Affirmation of the Day:

_____

Thoughts/feelings to let go of:

_____
_____
_____

This is your reminder to:

Change your phrases from "I can't" "It's too hard" or "I'm not good enough" to:

"I CAN" and "I WILL"
"I AM learning"
"I AM becoming"
"I AM unstoppable"
"I AM passionate"
"I AM capable"
"I AM worthy"
"I AM going to succeed"
"I AM PHENOMENAL"

See how these words make you feel?
start believing in **YOU**.
Take action and start showing up for
yourself EVERYDAY!!!

YOU CAN
DO iT!

Week 8

This week's self-care ritual:

_____
_____
_____
_____

This week I aspire to:

_____
_____
_____
_____

Something that made me smile this week?

_____
_____
_____
_____

What do I LOVE most about myself this week?

3 Things I am Grateful for:

1-

_____

_____

_____

_____

2-

_____

_____

_____

_____

3-

_____

_____

_____

_____

Positive Affirmation of the Day:

_____

Thoughts/feelings to let go of:

_____

_____

_____

Date: / /
3 Things I am Grateful for:

1-

_____
_____
_____
_____

2-

_____
_____
_____
_____

3-

_____
_____
_____
_____

Positive Affirmation of the Day:

_____

Thoughts/feelings to let go of:

_____
_____
_____

3 Things I am Grateful for:

1-

_____

_____

_____

_____

2-

_____

_____

_____

_____

3-

_____

_____

_____

_____

Positive Affirmation of the Day:

_____

Thoughts/feelings to let go of:

_____

_____

_____

Date: / /
3 Things I am Grateful for:

1-

_____

_____

_____

_____

2-

_____

_____

_____

_____

3-

_____

_____

_____

_____

Positive Affirmation of the Day:

_____

Thoughts/feelings to let go of:

_____

_____

_____

Date: / /

3 Things I am Grateful for:

1-

_____

_____

_____

_____

2-

_____

_____

_____

_____

3-

_____

_____

_____

_____

Positive Affirmation of the Day:

_____

Thoughts/feelings to let go of:

_____

_____

_____

Date: / /

3 Things I am Grateful for:

1-

_____

_____

_____

_____

2-

_____

_____

_____

_____

3-

_____

_____

_____

_____

Positive Affirmation of the Day:

_____

Thoughts/feelings to let go of:

_____

_____

_____

Fun Fact:

Did you know that taking a **COLD SHOWER** 2-3 times
a week can improve your health & well-being?

Here are some of the benefits:

- Boost your immune system
- Helps improve your metabolism
- Increased endorphins (may help to relieve depression & anxiety)
- Improves circulation
- Improves hair and skin
- Increases willpower

Want to feel more awake and alert?
Start your day right!

Now I'm not saying it's going to be easy,
BUT start with normal warm water,
then switch to cold at the end. Allow your body
to get used to the cold, take deep breaths to
boost oxygen flow.
Overtime the process will become easier.

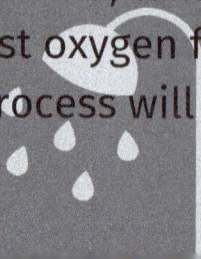

__Week 9__

This week's self-care ritual:

_____

_____

_____

_____

This week I aspire to:

_____

_____

_____

_____

What memory am I most fond of?

_____

_____

_____

_____

What do I LOVE most about myself this week?

Date: / /

3 Things I am Grateful for:

1-

_____

_____

_____

_____

2-

_____

_____

_____

3-

_____

_____

_____

_____

Positive Affirmation of the Day:

_____

Thoughts/feelings to let go of:

_____

_____

_____

Date: /   /

3 Things I am Grateful for:

1-

_____
_____
_____
_____

2-

_____
_____
_____
_____

3-

_____
_____
_____
_____

Positive Affirmation of the Day:

_____

Thoughts/feelings to let go of:

_____
_____
_____

3 Things I am Grateful for:

1-

_____
_____
_____
_____

2-

_____
_____
_____
_____

3-

_____
_____
_____
_____

Positive Affirmation of the Day:

_____

Thoughts/feelings to let go of:

_____
_____
_____

Date: / /

3 Things I am Grateful for:

1-

_____

_____

_____

_____

2-

_____

_____

_____

_____

3-

_____

_____

_____

_____

Positive Affirmation of the Day:

_____

Thoughts/feelings to let go of:

_____

_____

3 Things I am Grateful for:

1-

_____
_____
_____
_____

2-

_____
_____
_____
_____

3-

_____
_____
_____
_____

Positive Affirmation of the Day:

_____

Thoughts/feelings to let go of:

_____
_____
_____

3 Things I am Grateful for:

1-

_____

_____

_____

_____

2-

_____

_____

_____

_____

3-

_____

_____

_____

_____

Positive Affirmation of the Day:

_____

Thoughts/feelings to let go of:

_____

_____

_____

Date: / /

3 Things I am Grateful for:

1-

_____

_____

_____

_____

2-

_____

_____

_____

_____

3-

_____

_____

_____

_____

Positive Affirmation of the Day:

_____

Thoughts/feelings to let go of:

_____

_____

_____

"Fall in love with yourself, with life, and then with whoever you want"

-Frida Kahlo

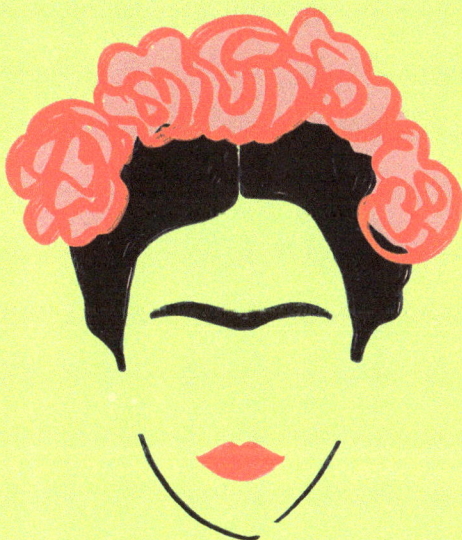

Week 10

This week's self-care ritual:

_____

_____

_____

_____

This week I aspire to:

_____

_____

_____

_____

What is one thing I appreciate about my life, that
I am creating for myself?

_____

_____

_____

_____

What do I LOVE most about myself this week?

Date: / /

3 Things I am Grateful for:

1-

_____
_____
_____
_____

2-

_____
_____
_____
_____

3-

_____
_____
_____
_____

Positive Affirmation of the Day:

_____

Thoughts/feelings to let go of:

_____
_____
_____

Date: /   /
3 Things I am Grateful for:

1-

2-

3-

Positive Affirmation of the Day:

Thoughts/feelings to let go of:

Date: / /
3 Things I am Grateful for:

1-

_____
_____
_____
_____

2-

_____
_____
_____
_____

3-

_____
_____
_____
_____

Positive Affirmation of the Day:

_____

Thoughts/feelings to let go of:

_____
_____
_____

Date: /   /

3 Things I am Grateful for:

1-

_____
_____
_____
_____

2-

_____
_____
_____
_____

3-

_____
_____
_____
_____

Positive Affirmation of the Day:

_____

Thoughts/feelings to let go of:

_____
_____
_____

Date: / /

3 Things I am Grateful for:

1-

_____
_____
_____
_____

2-

_____
_____
_____
_____

3-

_____
_____
_____
_____

Positive Affirmation of the Day:

_____

Thoughts/feelings to let go of:

_____
_____
_____

Date: / /
3 Things I am Grateful for:

1-

_____

_____

_____

_____

2-

_____

_____

_____

_____

3-

_____

_____

_____

_____

Positive Affirmation of the Day:

_____

Thoughts/feelings to let go of:

_____

_____

_____

Date: /   /

3 Things I am Grateful for:

1-

_____
_____
_____
_____

2-

_____
_____
_____
_____

3-

_____
_____
_____
_____

Positive Affirmation of the Day:

_____

Thoughts/feelings to let go of:

_____
_____
_____

WHEN YOU CHANGE THE WAY YOU LOOK AT THINGS, THE THINGS YOU LOOK AT CHANGE.

-Wayne Dyer

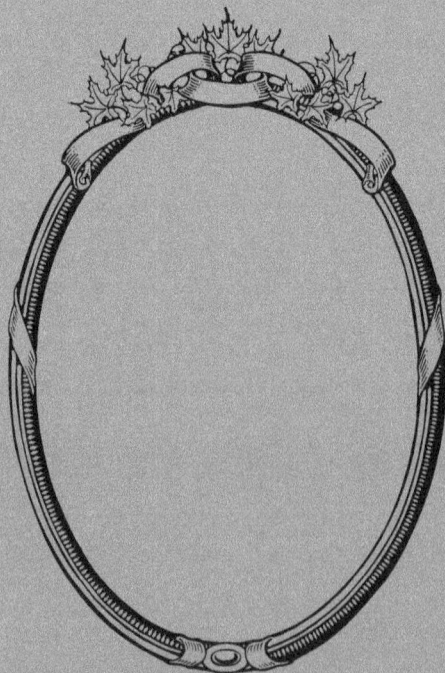

<u>Week 11</u>

This week's self-care ritual:

_____
_____
_____
_____

This week I aspire to:

_____
_____
_____
_____

I am most myself when I am with?

_____
_____
_____
_____

What do I LOVE most about myself this week?

_____

3 Things I am Grateful for:

1-

_____
_____
_____
_____

2-

_____
_____
_____
_____

3-

_____
_____
_____
_____

Positive Affirmation of the Day:

_____

Thoughts/feelings to let go of:

_____
_____
_____

Date: /   /

3 Things I am Grateful for:

1-

_____

_____

_____

_____

2-

_____

_____

_____

_____

3-

_____

_____

_____

_____

Positive Affirmation of the Day:

_____

Thoughts/feelings to let go of:

_____

_____

_____

3 Things I am Grateful for:

1-

_____

_____

_____

_____

2-

_____

_____

_____

_____

3-

_____

_____

_____

_____

Positive Affirmation of the Day:

_____

Thoughts/feelings to let go of:

_____

_____

_____

Date: /   /

3 Things I am Grateful for:

1-

_____

_____

_____

_____

2-

_____

_____

_____

_____

3-

_____

_____

_____

_____

Positive Affirmation of the Day:

_____

Thoughts/feelings to let go of:

_____

_____

_____

Date: /   /

3 Things I am Grateful for:

1-

_____
_____
_____
_____

2-

_____
_____
_____
_____

3-

_____
_____
_____
_____

Positive Affirmation of the Day:

_____

Thoughts/feelings to let go of:

_____
_____
_____

Date: /   /
3 Things I am Grateful for:

1-

_____
_____
_____
_____

2-

_____
_____
_____
_____

3-

_____
_____
_____
_____

Positive Affirmation of the Day:

_____

Thoughts/feelings to let go of:

_____
_____
_____

3 Things I am Grateful for:

1-

_____
_____
_____
_____

2-

_____
_____
_____
_____

3-

_____
_____
_____
_____

Positive Affirmation of the Day:

_____

Thoughts/feelings to let go of:

_____
_____
_____

Earthing/Grounding!

Now it may sound kind of funny BUT did you know that getting direct skin contact with the surface of the earth, whether it be with your hands or bare feet, allows the earth's electrons to transfer into the body, giving you direct energy from the earth.
I know crazy right, and how simple, by connecting to the Earth's natural energy, bringing your body back into a state of balance. Earthing also known as grounding, has many health benefits:

-Reduce inflammation
-Improves sleep
-Promotes calmness
-Boost antioxidants
-Improved circulation
-Increased energy levels
-Eliminates the excess of free radicals- which can slow the ageing process down.
-Normalises cortisol levels - improving hormone levels/stress levels.

By spending 10-30minutes a day of earthing you can really begin to reap the benefits and the best part is - it's FREE!

Week 12

This week's self-care ritual:

_____

_____

_____

_____

This week I aspire to:

_____

_____

_____

_____

When things don't go to plan what are some
things I can do to keep moving forward?

_____

_____

_____

_____

What do I LOVE most about myself this week?

Date: / /

3 Things I am Grateful for:

1-

_____

_____

_____

_____

2-

_____

_____

_____

_____

3-

_____

_____

_____

_____

Positive Affirmation of the Day:

_____

Thoughts/feelings to let go of:

_____

_____

_____

Date: /   /

3 Things I am Grateful for:

1-

_____
_____
_____
_____

2-

_____
_____
_____
_____

3-

_____
_____
_____
_____

Positive Affirmation of the Day:

_____

Thoughts/feelings to let go of:

_____
_____
_____

Date: / /
3 Things I am Grateful for:

1-

_____
_____
_____
_____

2-

_____
_____
_____
_____

3-

_____
_____
_____
_____

Positive Affirmation of the Day:

_____

Thoughts/feelings to let go of:

_____
_____
_____

Date: /   /

3 Things I am Grateful for:

1-

_____

_____

_____

_____

2-

_____

_____

_____

_____

3-

_____

_____

_____

_____

Positive Affirmation of the Day:

_____

Thoughts/feelings to let go of:

_____

_____

_____

Date: / /
3 Things I am Grateful for:

1-

_____

_____

_____

_____

2-

_____

_____

_____

_____

3-

_____

_____

_____

_____

Positive Affirmation of the Day:

_____

Thoughts/feelings to let go of:

_____

_____

_____

Date: /   /
3 Things I am Grateful for:

1-

_____

_____

_____

_____

2-

_____

_____

_____

_____

3-

_____

_____

_____

_____

Positive Affirmation of the Day:

_____

Thoughts/feelings to let go of:

_____

_____

_____

Date: / /

3 Things I am Grateful for:

1-

_____
_____
_____
_____

2-

_____
_____
_____
_____

3-

_____
_____
_____
_____

Positive Affirmation of the Day:

_____

Thoughts/feelings to let go of:

_____
_____
_____

DO THINGS FROM LOVE

NOT

FOR LOVE

-unknown

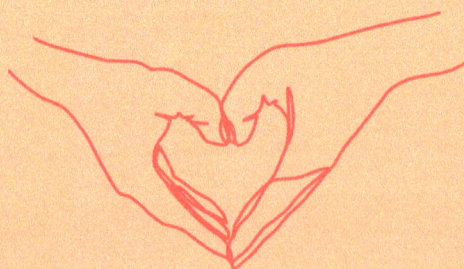

Week 13

This week's self-care ritual:

_____
_____
_____
_____

This week I aspire to:

_____
_____
_____
_____

What are my core values when it comes to
relationships?

_____
_____
_____
_____

What do I LOVE most about myself this week?

Date: / /
3 Things I am Grateful for:

1-

_____
_____
_____
_____

2-

_____
_____
_____
_____

3-

_____
_____
_____
_____

Positive Affirmation of the Day:

_____

Thoughts/feelings to let go of:

_____
_____
_____

3 Things I am Grateful for:

1-

_____

_____

_____

_____

2-

_____

_____

_____

_____

3-

_____

_____

_____

_____

Positive Affirmation of the Day:

_____

Thoughts/feelings to let go of:

_____

_____

_____

Date: / /

3 Things I am Grateful for:

1-

_____

_____

_____

_____

2-

_____

_____

_____

_____

3-

_____

_____

_____

_____

Positive Affirmation of the Day:

_____

Thoughts/feelings to let go of:

_____

_____

_____

Date: /   /

3 Things I am Grateful for:

1-

_____

_____

_____

_____

2-

_____

_____

_____

_____

3-

_____

_____

_____

_____

Positive Affirmation of the Day:

_____

Thoughts/feelings to let go of:

_____

_____

_____

Date: / /

3 Things I am Grateful for:

1-

_____

_____

_____

_____

2-

_____

_____

_____

_____

3-

_____

_____

_____

_____

Positive Affirmation of the Day:

_____

Thoughts/feelings to let go of:

_____

_____

_____

Date: / /

3 Things I am Grateful for:

1-

_____

_____

_____

_____

2-

_____

_____

_____

_____

3-

_____

_____

_____

_____

Positive Affirmation of the Day:

_____

Thoughts/feelings to let go of:

_____

_____

_____

Date: /   /

3 Things I am Grateful for:

1-

_____

_____

_____

_____

2-

_____

_____

_____

_____

3-

_____

_____

_____

_____

Positive Affirmation of the Day:

_____

Thoughts/feelings to let go of:

_____

_____

_____

Self-Talk Exercise: Changing the Narrative - Reframe, Retrain!

Do you agree that we are our own biggest critics? Sometimes we don't even notice when our internal critical voice presents itself.

Have you ever stopped and thought to yourself whilst your inner critic was present, would I speak to a loved one like this?

For example, you're having difficulty learning a new skill, so you begin to put yourself down, "I suck at this, I'm never going to get it".

Now think, if you saw a loved one struggling, would you say to them, that they suck and that they're never going to get it?

I'm guessing the answer is NO.

So, why is it ok to talk to ourselves in this manner? The answer is plain and simple, it is NOT ok.

So, the next time you find your inner critic present itself, think about the current situation and how you might respond to a loved one.

Reframe the language you use and try responding to the situation in the same way you would to a loved one and see how this makes you feel?

At the end of the day, we are a product of our own thoughts & what we CHOOSE to believe!

so, ALWAYS choose to be kind to yourself!

AND always back yourself!

<u>Week 14</u>

This week's self-care ritual:

_____

_____

_____

_____

This week I aspire to:

_____

_____

_____

_____

What body part am I most grateful for?

_____

_____

_____

_____

What do I LOVE most about myself this week?

Date: /   /

3 Things I am Grateful for:

1-

_____
_____
_____
_____

2-

_____
_____
_____
_____

3-

_____
_____
_____
_____

Positive Affirmation of the Day:

_____

Thoughts/feelings to let go of:

_____
_____
_____

Date: /   /

3 Things I am Grateful for:

1-

_____

_____

_____

_____

2-

_____

_____

_____

_____

3-

_____

_____

_____

_____

Positive Affirmation of the Day:

_____

Thoughts/feelings to let go of:

_____

_____

_____

Date: / /

3 Things I am Grateful for:

1-

_____
_____
_____
_____

2-

_____
_____
_____
_____

3-

_____
_____
_____
_____

Positive Affirmation of the Day:

_____

Thoughts/feelings to let go of:

_____
_____
_____

Date: / /
3 Things I am Grateful for:

1-

_____
_____
_____
_____

2-

_____
_____
_____
_____

3-

_____
_____
_____
_____

Positive Affirmation of the Day:

_____

Thoughts/feelings to let go of:

_____
_____
_____

Date: /   /

3 Things I am Grateful for:

1-

_____

_____

_____

_____

2-

_____

_____

_____

_____

3-

_____

_____

_____

_____

Positive Affirmation of the Day:

_____

Thoughts/feelings to let go of:

_____

_____

_____

Date: / /
3 Things I am Grateful for:

1-

_____

_____

_____

_____

2-

_____

_____

_____

_____

3-

_____

_____

_____

_____

Positive Affirmation of the Day:

_____

Thoughts/feelings to let go of:

_____

_____

_____

Date: / /
3 Things I am Grateful for:

1-

_____
_____
_____
_____

2-

_____
_____
_____
_____

3-

_____
_____
_____
_____

Positive Affirmation of the Day:

_____

Thoughts/feelings to let go of:

_____
_____
_____

If you can imagine it,
YOU can achieve it.
If you can dream it,
YOU can become it.

-William Arthur Ward

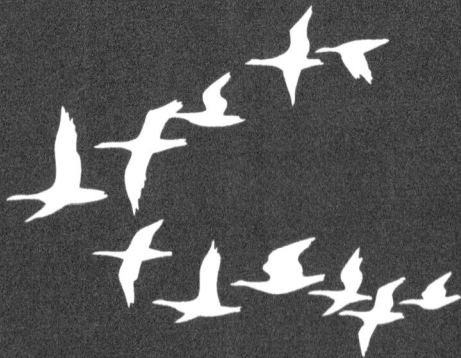

<u>Week 15</u>

This week's self-care ritual:

_____
_____
_____
_____

This week I aspire to:

_____
_____
_____
_____

Name 3 good deeds I can do for others this week?
AND do them.

_____
_____
_____
_____

What do I LOVE most about myself this week?

3 Things I am Grateful for:

1-

_____

_____

_____

_____

2-

_____

_____

_____

_____

3-

_____

_____

_____

_____

Positive Affirmation of the Day:

_____

Thoughts/feelings to let go of:

_____

_____

_____

Date: / /
3 Things I am Grateful for:

1-

_____
_____
_____
_____

2-

_____
_____
_____
_____

3-

_____
_____
_____
_____

Positive Affirmation of the Day:

_____

Thoughts/feelings to let go of:

_____
_____
_____

Date: / /

3 Things I am Grateful for:

1-

_____
_____
_____
_____

2-

_____
_____
_____
_____

3-

_____
_____
_____
_____

Positive Affirmation of the Day:

_____

Thoughts/feelings to let go of:

_____
_____
_____

Date: / /

3 Things I am Grateful for:

1-

_____

_____

_____

_____

2-

_____

_____

_____

_____

3-

_____

_____

_____

_____

Positive Affirmation of the Day:

_____

Thoughts/feelings to let go of:

_____

_____

_____

Date: / /

3 Things I am Grateful for:

1-

_____
_____
_____
_____

2-

_____
_____
_____
_____

3-

_____
_____
_____
_____

Positive Affirmation of the Day:

_____

Thoughts/feelings to let go of:

_____
_____
_____

3 Things I am Grateful for:

1-

_____

_____

_____

_____

2-

_____

_____

_____

_____

3-

_____

_____

_____

_____

Positive Affirmation of the Day:

_____

Thoughts/feelings to let go of:

_____

_____

_____

Date: /   /

3 Things I am Grateful for:

1-

_____
_____
_____
_____

2-

_____
_____
_____
_____

3-

_____
_____
_____
_____

Positive Affirmation of the Day:

_____

Thoughts/feelings to let go of:

_____
_____
_____

Let's talk about Dopamine
What is dopamine?

A chemical released in the brain that makes you feel good- the pleasure and reward center.

Ever wonder why junk food is so addictive? This is because it triggers our brains 'reward zone' every time you eat sugar it releases dopamine - which is why junk food can become so addictive. So, it's not necessarily the food that we are craving more so it's the hit of dopamine that leaves us wanting more, forming unhealthy habits, BUT did you know that there are many other healthy foods that can give you the same release of dopamine:

-Pumpkin seeds & sesame seeds
-Legumes
-Almonds & peanuts
-Apples, bananas & berries
-Avocados & spinach
-Eggs & dairy products
-Fish & poultry
-Green tea
-Dark chocolate

Just to name a few.
Exercise, music & meditation can also release dopamine.

<u>Week 16</u>

This week's self-care ritual:

_____

_____

_____

_____

This week I aspire to:

_____

_____

_____

_____

What is something I am better at this week than last week?

_____

_____

_____

_____

What do I LOVE most about myself this week?

Date: / /

3 Things I am Grateful for:

1-

_____
_____
_____
_____

2-

_____
_____
_____
_____

3-

_____
_____
_____
_____

Positive Affirmation of the Day:

_____

Thoughts/feelings to let go of:

_____
_____
_____

Date: /   /

3 Things I am Grateful for:

1-

2-

3-

Positive Affirmation of the Day:

Thoughts/feelings to let go of:

Date: /   /

3 Things I am Grateful for:

1-

_____
_____
_____
_____

2-

_____
_____
_____
_____

3-

_____
_____
_____
_____

Positive Affirmation of the Day:

_____

Thoughts/feelings to let go of:

_____
_____
_____

Date: / /
3 Things I am Grateful for:

1-

_____
_____
_____
_____

2-

_____
_____
_____
_____

3-

_____
_____
_____
_____

Positive Affirmation of the Day:

_____

Thoughts/feelings to let go of:

_____
_____
_____

Date: / /

3 Things I am Grateful for:

1-

_____
_____
_____
_____

2-

_____
_____
_____
_____

3-

_____
_____
_____
_____

Positive Affirmation of the Day:

_____

Thoughts/feelings to let go of:

_____
_____
_____

Date: / /

3 Things I am Grateful for:

1-

_____
_____
_____
_____

2-

_____
_____
_____
_____

3-

_____
_____
_____
_____

Positive Affirmation of the Day:

_____

Thoughts/feelings to let go of:

_____
_____
_____

Date: /   /

3 Things I am Grateful for:

1-

_____
_____
_____
_____

2-

_____
_____
_____
_____

3-

_____
_____
_____
_____

Positive Affirmation of the Day:

_____

Thoughts/feelings to let go of:

_____
_____
_____

To be vulnerable isn't always something that comes easy, BUT the more we stay in our comfort zone the more likely we are to miss out on opportunities in reaching our true potential.

So, I challenge you to step outside of your comfort zone, get vulnerable. You'll be surprised at how strong and resilient you can be!
This week I invite you to do something you wouldn't usually do. See how this makes you feel!
Invigorated? Scared? Excited?
What comes up for you?

The more you test the waters the easier it becomes! Start believing in the power of YOU today and every day and watch the magic unfold!
YOU'VE GOT THIS!

I'm not saying it's going to be easy and yes things may not go to plan BUT take the lesson and continue to strive for excellence, as the saying goes "Rome wasn't built in a day".

__Week 17__

This week's self-care ritual:

_____

_____

_____

_____

This week I aspire to:

_____

_____

_____

_____

What day of the week do I look forward to most?
why?

_____

_____

_____

_____

What do I LOVE most about myself this week?

3 Things I am Grateful for:

1-

_____
_____
_____
_____

2-

_____
_____
_____
_____

3-

_____
_____
_____
_____

Positive Affirmation of the Day:

_____

Thoughts/feelings to let go of:

_____
_____
_____

Date: /   /

3 Things I am Grateful for:

1-

_____
_____
_____
_____

2-

_____
_____
_____
_____

3-

_____
_____
_____
_____

Positive Affirmation of the Day:

_____

Thoughts/feelings to let go of:

_____
_____
_____

Date: /   /

3 Things I am Grateful for:

1-

_____

_____

_____

_____

2-

_____

_____

_____

_____

3-

_____

_____

_____

_____

Positive Affirmation of the Day:

_____

Thoughts/feelings to let go of:

_____

_____

_____

Date: /   /

3 Things I am Grateful for:

1-

_____

_____

_____

_____

2-

_____

_____

_____

_____

3-

_____

_____

_____

_____

Positive Affirmation of the Day:

_____

Thoughts/feelings to let go of:

_____

_____

_____

Date: /   /

3 Things I am Grateful for:

1-

_____

_____

_____

_____

2-

_____

_____

_____

_____

3-

_____

_____

_____

_____

Positive Affirmation of the Day:

_____

Thoughts/feelings to let go of:

_____

_____

_____

Date: /   /

3 Things I am Grateful for:

1-

_____

_____

_____

_____

2-

_____

_____

_____

_____

3-

_____

_____

_____

_____

Positive Affirmation of the Day:

_____

Thoughts/feelings to let go of:

_____

_____

_____

3 Things I am Grateful for:

1-

_____

_____

_____

_____

2-

_____

_____

_____

_____

3-

_____

_____

_____

_____

Positive Affirmation of the Day:

_____

Thoughts/feelings to let go of:

_____

_____

_____

Immune Boosting Soup

Ingredients:

- 500mls chicken bone broth
- 500g chicken mince
- 2-3 stalks of celery chopped
- 1 large carrot peeled & chopped
- 1 cup of spinach
- 1/2 red onion
- 1 cup of kale
- 1 zucchini chopped
- 1/2 red capsicum diced
- Handful of mushrooms chopped
- 2 cloves garlic roughly chopped
- 2-3cm fresh ginger grated or roughly chopped
- 1 fresh chili chopped
- 1 tsp ground turmeric
- Juice from 1 lemon
- Generous splash of soy sauce
- Generous splash of sesame oil
- Handful of fresh coriander chopped (optional)

Packed with antioxidants, tons of nutrients & minerals & has anti-inflammatory benefits.

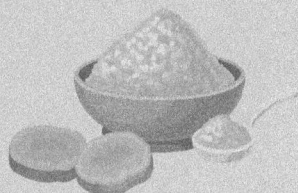

Method:

1- Heat olive oil in pot over medium heat. Add carrots, celery, onion, 1/2 of the garlic, 1/2 of ginger and chili, sauté until vegetables are softened.

2- Add Chicken and cook through.

3- In another pot add chicken bone broth, mushrooms, remaining ginger & garlic (top up with 500ml of boiling water.

4- Once chicken is cooked through add your capsicum, zucchini, spinach, kale & broth mixture.

5 - Continue to cook on low, add lemon juice, soy sauce & sesame oil, along with coriander, season with salt and pepper.

Week 18

This week's self-care ritual:

_____
_____
_____
_____

This week I aspire to:

_____
_____
_____
_____

What makes me a good friend?

_____
_____
_____
_____

What do I LOVE most about myself this week?

Date: /   /

3 Things I am Grateful for:

1-

_____
_____
_____
_____

2-

_____
_____
_____
_____

3-

_____
_____
_____
_____

Positive Affirmation of the Day:

_____

Thoughts/feelings to let go of:

_____
_____
_____

Date: /   /

3 Things I am Grateful for:

1-

_____
_____
_____
_____

2-

_____
_____
_____
_____

3-

_____
_____
_____
_____

Positive Affirmation of the Day:

_____

Thoughts/feelings to let go of:

_____
_____
_____

Date: /   /

3 Things I am Grateful for:

1-

_____
_____
_____
_____

2-

_____
_____
_____
_____

3-

_____
_____
_____
_____

Positive Affirmation of the Day:

_____

Thoughts/feelings to let go of:

_____
_____
_____

3 Things I am Grateful for:

1-

_____

_____

_____

_____

2-

_____

_____

_____

_____

3-

_____

_____

_____

_____

Positive Affirmation of the Day:

_____

Thoughts/feelings to let go of:

_____

_____

_____

Date: / /

3 Things I am Grateful for:

1-

_____
_____
_____
_____

2-

_____
_____
_____
_____

3-

_____
_____
_____
_____

Positive Affirmation of the Day:

_____

Thoughts/feelings to let go of:

_____
_____
_____

Date: / /
3 Things I am Grateful for:

1-

_____
_____
_____
_____

2-

_____
_____
_____
_____

3-

_____
_____
_____
_____

Positive Affirmation of the Day:

_____

Thoughts/feelings to let go of:

_____
_____
_____

Date: / /

3 Things I am Grateful for:

1-

_____
_____
_____
_____

2-

_____
_____
_____
_____

3-

_____
_____
_____
_____

Positive Affirmation of the Day:

_____

Thoughts/feelings to let go of:

_____
_____
_____

Today I invite you to let go of who you think you're supposed to be and start truly embracing your own authentic self!

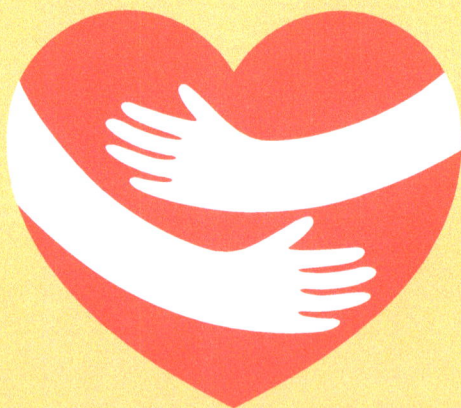

Week 19

This week's self-care ritual:

_____
_____
_____
_____

This week I aspire to:

_____
_____
_____
_____

What makes me UNIQUE?

_____
_____
_____
_____

What do I LOVE most about myself this week?

3 Things I am Grateful for:

1-

_____

_____

_____

_____

2-

_____

_____

_____

_____

3-

_____

_____

_____

_____

Positive Affirmation of the Day:

_____

Thoughts/feelings to let go of:

_____

_____

_____

Date: /   /

3 Things I am Grateful for:

1-

_____
_____
_____
_____

2-

_____
_____
_____
_____

3-

_____
_____
_____
_____

Positive Affirmation of the Day:

_____

Thoughts/feelings to let go of:

_____
_____
_____

Date: /   /

3 Things I am Grateful for:

1-

_____

_____

_____

_____

2-

_____

_____

_____

_____

3-

_____

_____

_____

_____

Positive Affirmation of the Day:

_____

Thoughts/feelings to let go of:

_____

_____

_____

Date: / /
3 Things I am Grateful for:

1-

_____
_____
_____
_____

2-

_____
_____
_____
_____

3-

_____
_____
_____
_____

Positive Affirmation of the Day:

_____

Thoughts/feelings to let go of:

_____
_____
_____

Date: / /

3 Things I am Grateful for:

1-

_____

_____

_____

_____

2-

_____

_____

_____

_____

3-

_____

_____

_____

_____

Positive Affirmation of the Day:

_____

Thoughts/feelings to let go of:

_____

_____

_____

Date: / /
3 Things I am Grateful for:

1-

_____
_____
_____
_____

2-

_____
_____
_____
_____

3-

_____
_____
_____
_____

Positive Affirmation of the Day:

_____

Thoughts/feelings to let go of:

_____
_____
_____

Date: /   /

3 Things I am Grateful for:

1-

2-

3-

Positive Affirmation of the Day:

Thoughts/feelings to let go of:

SLEEP!

It's time we spoke about sleep.

Adults need 7 to 9 hours of sleep per night.
Below are some tips on how to support quality sleep which will then support your overall health and wellbeing. Sleep improves mood, helps you feel more energised, improves memory, concentration & productivity, reduces the risk of illness and boosts your immune system. Efficient sleep also plays a part in weight management.

1 hour before bed is the ideal time to start your sleep rituals:

- Set a consistent sleep and wake time to help the body keep an internal clock and will train the brain to naturally feel tired when it's bedtime.
- Expose yourself to morning sunlight.
- Exercise throughout the day to support better sleep quality, (try to avoid exercise too late in the day to allow your body time to rest before bed).
- Avoid screen time at least 30mintues before bed and ensure your sleep environment is cool, dark and quiet.
- Avoid caffeinated drinks after 4:00pm.
- Don't go to bed on a full or hungry stomach.
- Avoid alcohol before bed - try drinking herbal tea like Chamomile tea.
- Meditation, stretching & breathwork can also support a healthy sleep routine - allowing physical/mental tensions from the day to melt away, evoking the relaxation response in the body and producing melatonin - the sleep hormone.

And of course, practice GRATITUDE every night before you go to sleep and when you wake.

Week 20

This week's self-care ritual:

_____
_____
_____
_____

This week I aspire to:

_____
_____
_____
_____

When do I feel most confident?

_____
_____
_____
_____

What do I LOVE most about myself this week?

Date: /   /

3 Things I am Grateful for:

1-

_____
_____
_____
_____

2-

_____
_____
_____
_____

3-

_____
_____
_____
_____

Positive Affirmation of the Day:

_____

Thoughts/feelings to let go of:

_____
_____
_____

Date: /   /

3 Things I am Grateful for:

1-

_____

_____

_____

_____

2-

_____

_____

_____

_____

3-

_____

_____

_____

_____

Positive Affirmation of the Day:

_____

Thoughts/feelings to let go of:

_____

_____

_____

3 Things I am Grateful for:

1-

_____
_____
_____
_____

2-

_____
_____
_____
_____

3-

_____
_____
_____
_____

Positive Affirmation of the Day:

_____

Thoughts/feelings to let go of:

_____
_____
_____

Date: /   /

3 Things I am Grateful for:

1-

_____

_____

_____

_____

2-

_____

_____

_____

_____

3-

_____

_____

_____

_____

Positive Affirmation of the Day:

_____

Thoughts/feelings to let go of:

_____

_____

_____

Date: / /

3 Things I am Grateful for:

1-

_____
_____
_____
_____

2-

_____
_____
_____
_____

3-

_____
_____
_____
_____

Positive Affirmation of the Day:

_____

Thoughts/feelings to let go of:

_____
_____
_____

3 Things I am Grateful for:

1-

2-

3-

Positive Affirmation of the Day:

Thoughts/feelings to let go of:

Date: /   /

3 Things I am Grateful for:

1-

_____
_____
_____
_____

2-

_____
_____
_____
_____

3-

_____
_____
_____
_____

Positive Affirmation of the Day:

_____

Thoughts/feelings to let go of:

_____
_____
_____

SLEEPY FOODS

Did you know that some foods and drinks have sleep promoting properties?

Some melatonin rich foods include:

- Tart cherries, grapes & cranberries
- Goji berries & bananas
- Milk & eggs
- Pistachios
- Fatty fish- Salmon
- Rice & oats
- Mushrooms

Other foods that improve sleep Include:

- Kiwi fruits - Vitamin C, folate & rich in serotonin.
- Avocados - Potassium increases serotonin production.
- Sweet potato - Potassium helps muscles relax.
- Legumes - Zinc helps improve sleep quality
- Spinach - High in magnesium.
- Chamomile tea - promotes sleep through antioxidant apigenin.

Week 21

This week's self-care ritual:

_____
_____
_____
_____

This week I aspire to:

_____
_____
_____
_____

If I could change one thing to make my life easier,
what would it be?

_____
_____
_____
_____

What do I LOVE most about myself this week?

Date: / /

3 Things I am Grateful for:

1-

_____
_____
_____
_____

2-

_____
_____
_____
_____

3-

_____
_____
_____
_____

Positive Affirmation of the Day:

_____

Thoughts/feelings to let go of:

_____
_____
_____

Date: / /

3 Things I am Grateful for:

1-

_____
_____
_____
_____

2-

_____
_____
_____
_____

3-

_____
_____
_____
_____

Positive Affirmation of the Day:

_____

Thoughts/feelings to let go of:

_____
_____
_____

3 Things I am Grateful for:

1-

_____
_____
_____
_____

2-

_____
_____
_____
_____

3-

_____
_____
_____
_____

Positive Affirmation of the Day:

_____

Thoughts/feelings to let go of:

_____
_____
_____

Date: /   /

3 Things I am Grateful for:

1-

_____
_____
_____
_____

2-

_____
_____
_____
_____

3-

_____
_____
_____
_____

Positive Affirmation of the Day:

_____

Thoughts/feelings to let go of:

_____
_____
_____

Date: / /

3 Things I am Grateful for:

1-

2-

3-

Positive Affirmation of the Day:

Thoughts/feelings to let go of:

Date: /   /

3 Things I am Grateful for:

1-

_____
_____
_____
_____

2-

_____
_____
_____
_____

3-

_____
_____
_____
_____

Positive Affirmation of the Day:

_____

Thoughts/feelings to let go of:

_____
_____
_____

Date: /   /

3 Things I am Grateful for:

1-

_____

_____

_____

_____

2-

_____

_____

_____

_____

3-

_____

_____

_____

_____

Positive Affirmation of the Day:

_____

Thoughts/feelings to let go of:

_____

_____

_____

The Power of Mindset!

Adopting a positive mindset is the gateway to possibilities, and the first step to any success - anything you want to achieve or create in life ALL comes back down to mindset.

YOU CAN DO ANYTHING YOU SET YOUR MIND TO!

If you spot it, you've got it, you just need to put in the groundwork. Invest time into your health & wellness, love yourself, believe in yourself, because when you create a happy, safe & loving place in your head, you are more likely to achieve your desired outcomes.

There is no failure only feedback.

Bring your good energy into the now, don't let your past define you. You have the power to recreate yourself, be the person you always wanted to be. Kindness doesn't cost a damn thing and to be kind to yourself is the
holy grail.

Often, we're too busy waiting for things to change, to get better, BUT reality check, things will not change, until you change your attitude, your mindset and you're willing to take action.

If you want to evolve, then stop making excuses. Prioritise the good things in your life, then identify the things that are no longer serving you, and let them go. And remember, we are all doing the best we can with the resources we have available.

YOU have the ability to create choice & wholeness. And remember to always stay GRATEFUL!

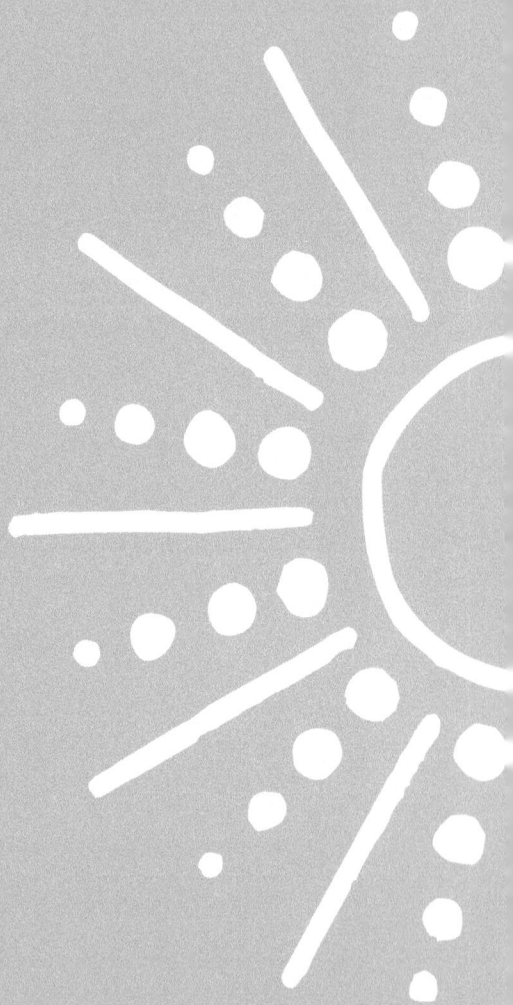

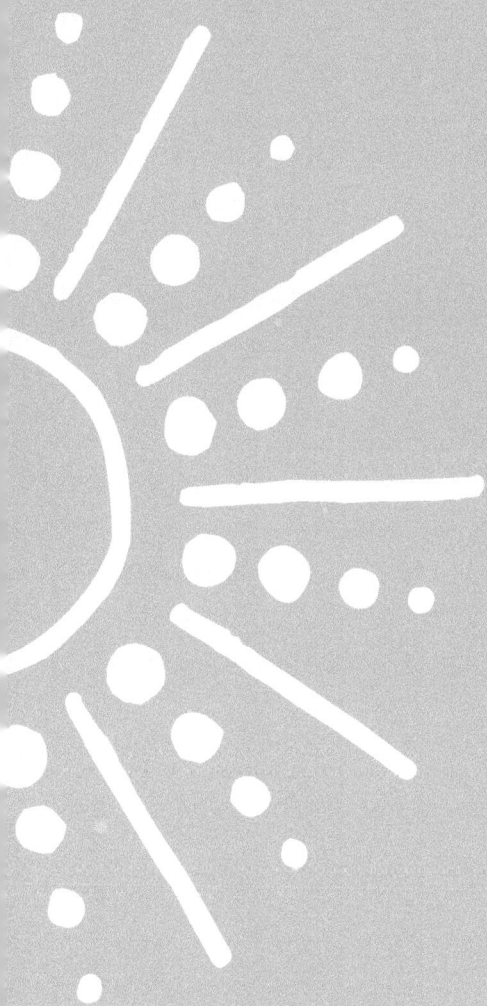

www.ingramcontent.com/pod-product-compliance
Lightning Source LLC
Chambersburg PA
CBHW041935260326
41914CB00010B/1313